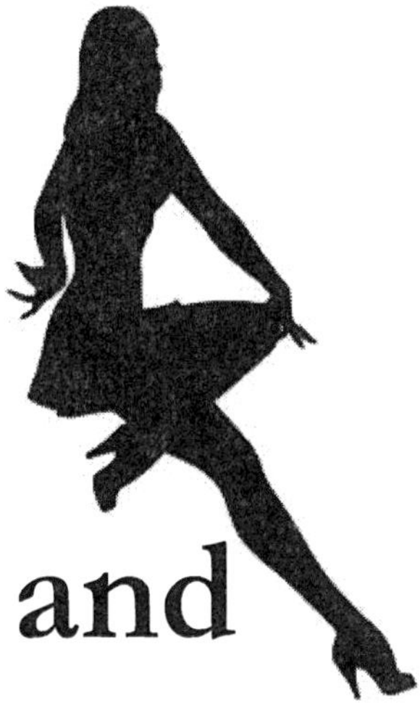

Foreplay, Roleplay and *Rounds*

Dr Sankalp Jain

Printed in India

ISBN: 978-93-5776-856-6
First Printing, 2023

THE WRITE ORDER

The Write Order
A division of Nasadiya Technologies Private Ltd.
Koramangala, Bangalore
Karnataka-560029
THE WRITE ORDER PUBLICATIONS.
www.thewriteorder.com

Edited by Anagha Somanakoppa
Book Cover designed by Sankhasubhro Nath
Publishing Consultant- Priyanka Lal

Contents

Preface

I began writing this book as a testimony to all the various cases and curiosities I have come across over the years. I felt the need to address some basic queries and questions that are being asked now more often than not in public spaces. Our society is slowly progressing towards inclusion for all, which brings us to a deeper issue of not having enough means to educate the masses about sex, as well as its related practices and behaviour.

At the same time understanding the responses of young generation towards gender identification, supporting gender neutral peers and understanding the sexual orientation of partners, is a mammoth task at hand.

I am writing this book as a memoir of all my various cases, keeping well in mind the patient's psychology associated with them and how can we learn and be more humane toward all kinds of people - straight, gay, queer, binary, non binary, transgender or asexual.

I hope my experiences will shine some light on the biggest taboo in our society i.e. sex.

About The Author

Born in a family of doctors, Dr Sankalp has always been the curious kid who spent a considerable amount of time with his Grandfather, whom he lovingly called 'Bawaji'. He wasn't any ordinary doctor, a Royal physician in his time, a brilliant doctor, an Ayurvedic medicine expert and a connoisseur of good food, his was a tall figure to match.

He laid the first foundation of medicine in Dr Sankalp's life and nurtured it till his very last breath.

His father, Dr A K Jain, a renowned Ayurvedic practitioner and philanthropist, continued the legacy, which is now a almost a century old and has been an active mentor in Dr Sankalp's life.

Dr Sankalp has erased the line between the old and new and is giving the best of both worlds to his patients, from both India and abroad. He himself being a modern medicine graduate, has brought together the time tested learnings of Ayurveda and the technological advances of modern medicine to treat his patients. He has a panel of doctors from both backgrounds, who along with his research team develop niche personalised treatments for each patient.

Chapter 1

Normalizing Sex

Let's talk about Sex, but how? It is considered taboo to talk about Sex, even with your partner or doctor. The concepts of equality, sexuality, freedom, liberty, and homosexuality are all prevalent in the 21st century, yet we never step on top of them. We feel uncomfortable and guilty after seeing a brief condom or sanitary pad advertisement. Why?

It is essential to identify why discussing Sex is odd and uncomfortable before delving further into the necessity to normalize the topic. Sex has historically been viewed as a personal act intended only to produce offspring. Sex naturally carries a tenuous thread of appropriateness and legality. The family is the beating heart of society, and it ensures that it continues to exist, propagates, teaches, and reteaches the morality of Sex through socialization. And that's how we are conditioned to believe Sex is sacred and can't be named out loud.

Sexuality is a lovely and empowering aspect of human nature, giving us excellent emotional and physical feelings. Being sexually active should not be stigmatized and isn't dishonourable or dirty. Our bodies are unique, complicated systems capable of incredible feats. Let's find out why normalizing Sex is essential:

- Every person on the planet was produced through sexual interaction. Given that humans would not exist without Sex, it is absurd to keep our sexual encounters with one another hidden. It's awful that women, even men discussing their sexual wants, make many others cringe. They should be encouraged and should feel free to discuss it openly. Discussions about sexual experiences with peers do not make you a bad person; they make you a better lover!
- The fundamental purpose of normalizing Sex is to remove the social constraints and preconceptions that are unfair to women, men, the LGBT community, and others. It will encourage them to embrace it because Sex is regular rather than making them feel bad. They will learn from this that there is more to the world than their sexual preferences and predefined boundaries.

Normalization of Sex will aid in disseminating sex education to the general public, which is critical. We're all aware of what Sex is. Yet how many of us are aware of its multi-layered complexity? Having sex conversations will help to raise awareness about the use of contraception and its dangers. It will also teach us that contraceptives are not a woman's burden but a personal choice. There are several sexually transmitted diseases, genital issues, and pregnancy issues to consider. In addition, women and men can suffer from several conditions that make Sex painful or unenjoyable. Being open and conversing about these topics allows people to feel less lonely.

The Health Resources and Services **Administration Advisory Committee on HIV, Viral Hepatitis, and STD Prevention and Treatment (CHAC) has developed the following definition of sexual health recommended for use in the U.S.:*Sexual health is a state of well-being about sexuality across the life span that involves physical, emotional, mental, social, and spiritual dimensions. Sexual health is an intrinsic element of human health and is based on a positive, equitable, and respectful approach to sexuality, relationships, and reproduction that is free of coercion, fear, discrimination, stigma, shame, and violence. It includes understanding the benefits, risks, and responsibilities of sexual behaviour; preventing and caring for disease and other adverse outcomes; and the possibility of fulfilling sexual relationships. Sexual health is impacted by socioeconomic and cultural contexts—including policies, practices, and services—that support healthy outcomes for individuals, families, and their communities.***

- In addition, if Sex is accepted as usual, people will be able to appreciate it for what it truly is: a sexual act of pleasure rather than reproduction. It will bust the belief that Sex is only used for reproduction. Children are a result of Sex, not the reason. Sex is intended to be pleasurable and enjoyable. A sex discussion will establish the actual necessity of Sex and educate us on the importance and rewards of participating in it.
- Normalizing Sex allows and makes us aware of using

correct labels like pansexual, asexual, etc., that are real, and awareness about these will make you a better human. And also, talking about Sex is not only limited to sharing experiences; it also makes us aware of sexuality identification, abuse in the marriage, puberty, and many more.

- Finally, by guaranteeing that no one is harmed or coerced into doing anything they don't want, you improve the world by normalizing sex discourse. Anytime you interact with people, in any manner, consent is essential. Our society has conditioned us to view Sex as taboo, but we have never been instructed on the importance of saying "no." We are never taught to draw boundaries because we have no idea where they should be. Normalizing sex-related communication will aid in understanding the importance of consent before engaging in sexual behaviors.

Even before birth, society gives us gender roles based on our genitals. A guy is expected to show masculinity and dominance, whereas a woman is expected to be meek and subservient. It's not like not talking about Sex only makes females the victim; men in society are also the victim because they fear rejection, body insecurities, and performance anxiety that makes them anxious. This rigidly binary framework paralyzes civilization and drags it farther into the pit of forgetfulness. One must start a discussion about this.

Sharing sexual experiences doesn't mean walking around screaming about Sex; it means sharing sexual experiences and problems with a friend, doctor, therapist, or anyone you want to share with. Sexuality is a multifaceted phenomenon having physical, psychological, and social aspects. The myths, labels, constructions, and binary thinking will be dismantled as sexuality becomes a regular topic of discourse.

Sex is natural. Sex is responsible for your existence. Don't feel vulnerable and uneasy. Embracing yourself and your body and having Sex without fear of judgment gives you confidence. Make the world what it promises to be: free. Be curious, ask questions, and consider your body's requirements. Be aware of your pain, joys, and overall body state.

Let's Normalize Sex!

Chapter 2
Myths & Facts

Sexuality is a basic instinct. Throughout childhood, youth, and maturity, everyone has views about sexuality and sexual conduct. The community's values, culture, and religion can all impact people's ideas about sexuality. Societies pass on patterns of thinking, opinions, and judgments to future generations that mature with time. We learn what is deemed proper or inappropriate regarding masculinity or femininity as we grow in a specific culture. Unfortunately, a significant portion of what we know and internalize is dysfunctional.

Women in this country have had roughly 50 years to reconsider their role in the world to organize and broaden the boundaries of female identity. Unfortunately, men have not yet had the opportunity. Parents overestimate their kids' physical prowess—how well they crawl—even before they can walk. We're instilling in them a performance-oriented masculinity focused on autonomy, silence, strength, fearlessness, and competition. This is toxic masculinity in action.

It's no secret that the way sex has been portrayed in

media, films, and perhaps even by some of your friends has been deceptive or, in some instances, outright inaccurate. Some sex expectations or false assumptions may impact your sex life or lead to intimacy issues, even if you are unaware. We live in an era when we know our bodies and are more in tune with our health than ever. Looking back at some of the sex-related claims made by "experts" over the years, it's worthwhile to differentiate fact from fantasy. This article discusses the myths passed on to us for ages and facts debunking those myths.

Myth: Size Matters!

Fact: Because porn and lack of sexual education have warped men's perceptions of penis size, many people decide to stop dating and fear making an intimate connection. There are many different sizes and styles of penises and testicles. Penises seem pretty diverse in size when they aren't erect, but their sizes are considerably more similar when they are. There is virtually no way for most guys to genuinely compare the size of their erect penis to that of other men. Nonetheless, the misconception remains; many men believe they must have a certain size to "measure up". It's no surprise they feel inadequate. An individual's level of enjoyment is unrelated to the size of his penis, and the level of pleasure his partner experiences is also unaffected.

Myth: Guys are constantly thinking or open to having sex

Fact: There are many situations when both men and women do not want to have sex and do not want to become "in the mood". Even though men enjoy sex, and even those who enjoy sex a lot, practically all men dislike sex. We all have days when we don't want to be sexually active.

Unfortunately, this stereotype might pressure males to perform even when they don't want to, putting extra strain on themselves. They may feel as if they cannot express their desire for sex. Guys must accept that they aren't sexual objects and should feel free to decline sexual advances. Men and their partners can both benefit from learning how to say no, making the sexual activity they do engage in that much more joyful.

There is so much variation in sexual urge that there is no such thing as "normal". Knowing that males experience many of the same problems as women—they're anxious, weary, and don't feel attractive—allows both parties to feel understood. A man's desire at any time does not predict his partner's beauty. Your desires will not always be aligned entirely—leave some wiggle room for each other to be out of the mood. Consider merely snuggling, as closeness does not require climax.

Myth: Men are not Virgin

Fact: Men occasionally lie about how much sex they have had or how frequently they have it. Although more than half of males have indeed engaged in sexual activity by the time they are 18, this percentage seems to be declining as more and more men put off having sex. In fact, by the time they turn 19, up to one in four guys had never engaged in sexual activity.

Myth: When a male ejaculates, sex is over

Fact: This does not have to be the case, and it should not be. When two people engage in sexual activity, it should continue until both participants are content and ready to quit. To ensure that the partners engage in enjoyable, comfortable, and satisfying activities, good sex requires constant communication and connection between the individuals.

Therefore, there is no reason why every sexual experience needs to entail climax or ejaculation. Men may have "blue balls" or "lover's nuts" if they have an erection but do not ejaculate; these are not dangerous circumstances. Men will feel discomfort, but developing the relationship and using creativity during sexual activity can result in better sex overall.

Myth: Masturbation indicates a lack of sexual interest in your partner

Fact: Masturbation is natural and is considered a crucial part of healthy sexual development. Masturbation is a healthy form of sexual expression, regardless of how frequently you do it or how long you've known your partner. Many people assume that having a spouse who masturbates in a relationship indicates that they are no longer sexually engaged in their mate. This is not the case, and no partner should interpret this behavior in any other way, at least not on its own.

Masturbation addiction, on the other hand, is a different issue. If you are suffering from a persistent and powerless masturbation addiction, seek assistance from a medical practitioner.

Myth: Men are only the sex initiator

Fact: This myth is so firmly embedded in sexual experiences that we rarely question it. As "nice girls" don't ask for or consent to sex throughout adolescence, men are burdened with the responsibility of courting and starting sexual activity. Yet this pattern of men pursuing sex and women gatekeeping does not simply stop when we reach adult relationships. For centuries, women have been persuaded that males only desire "one thing" and have been pushed to reject their advances. This puts much pressure on men, and sexual rejection is difficult for both genders, who experience unpleasant emotions such as low self-esteem and loss of interest in sex after rejection.

Sex is an act where two participants are needed, and both can be equally responsible for the initiation.

Myth: A woman's physical beauty primarily motivates men's desire

Fact: You've probably heard that physical clues arouse a man, and believing the myth that all men want women with perfect bodies completely ignores the depth of a man's sexuality. Women sometimes worry that their partners will lose interest in them as they gain weight or age. However, the truth is that men have various notions of beauty and are, in actuality, more drawn to a woman's confidence and her ability to let him know to connect.

Myth: Orgasm should be "mind-blowing"

Fact: If you've been surrounded by pulp novels and movies your entire life, you can have an unrealistic notion of what an orgasm is. The strength and character of orgasms vary, and they may experience various emotions from one situation to the next, which is very natural.

Why do we have such strong misconceptions about male sexuality?

The picture of men that we have is reinforced

everywhere. Men are portrayed in movies and songs as hounds continually looking for sex. Guys and women both talk about sex in this manner. The pressure of pseudo-masculinity claims about male sexuality being selfish and poisonous reinforced this. And we've become accustomed to the stereotype.

Are males more emotionally invested in sex than people realize?

Absolutely. Men's sexual desire is stimulated mainly by physical attractiveness, including lingerie, low-cut shirts, and high hemlines. Of course, this is correct. But we frequently overlook how important the emotional component is. Feeling connected and wanting to be close to his partner—not just physically—fuels a man's sexual desire. Men also want deep communication, a gentle stroke in hair, want to be vulnerable, and feel desire when they are heard by their spouse and are on the same page.

The condition frequently stigmatizes men with sexual inf, and humiliation is a major barrier to discussing the issue with healthcare providers. Men with PE believe they have little control over their ejaculation, and this loss of control is reflected in lower enjoyment of sexual intercourse. PE imposes an emotional and physical toll. Low self-esteem, fear, and emotions of humiliation and inferiority are all connected with premature ejaculation.

Prejudices and myths have specially conditioned male sexuality. These sexuality myths are ones that both men and women learn to believe. Internalizing these falsehoods can be harmful to men and their relationships. Here are just a handful of the negative consequences of internalizing these myths.

Distress and Anxiety

These male sexual desire myths create distress and anxiety. Guys who internalize the idea that men are always expected to want sex may experience self-consciousness when they aren't in the mood. These males may be anxious about being broken since they do not fit the perceived norm.

Develop Mistrust between Partners

Another issue with these fallacies is that women have been conditioned to distrust men in sexual situations. We are not referring to women who have legitimate reasons not to trust men (such as abuse, neglect, or other forms of abuse), and there are certainly guys who deserve their bad reputation. Many a lady has found it difficult to believe that her husband desires her for more than just sex, and many a husband has had to jump through hoops and focus solely on what his wife wants to prove that he is "not like other guys." The truth is that most guys (especially those you love and trust enough to marry) desire an emotional connection just as much as their female counterparts.

Men can't express their needs

Because of these myths, men do not have the space to ask for what they want. Being bound by a stereotype might make men feel as if there is a specific way they must act and react. This gives little room for males to experiment with their sexual desires. They frequently don't feel they have enough space to understand what they desire; are they attracted by physical characteristics or something more emotional? Are they desirous on their own, or do they react to what their spouse does? Most people fall between these two extremes, but many men are unaware they are special or can have a dynamic sex drive.

After knowing the myths and their effect on men's mental and physical health, it's time to understand how to deal with this situation. Here are a few strategies to dispel these myths in your personal and family interactions.

Leave space for an emotional connect

As there is no other way that feels "masculine," men frequently seek sex when they want to feel emotionally connected. Learn to recognize when your partner requests an emotional connection. We must respond appropriately when our partner makes a bid. It's also critical to make room for both couples to be emotionally vulnerable and seek a relationship. Let yourself feel your feelings, guys! And girls! be emotionally supportive of your partners. Believe that your partner wants you more than he wants sex.

Change the initiation game

Men face much pressure to be the initiator constantly. This works wonderfully for some couples. But, in other cases, it might result in a stressed-out husband and a dissatisfied wife. Therefore, ladies, try your hand at initiating. Be the one to initiate some foreplay. Find out what things make your hubby happy. Every couple will have a distinct initiating rhythm that works for them. But don't just assume that your hubby will always initiate sex!

Bring changes

In the same vein, don't be scared to experiment. Break harmful habits or discard items that are no longer useful. As previously stated, different stages of life will bring about variations in your sexual urge. Communication is essential, and have an open dialogue about what you enjoy and dislike. When you uncover something that is no longer working, learn to alter it without hesitation. Please don't be too hard on yourself; that item used to work, and now it doesn't! It says nothing about you as a lover or sexual person.

Learn about sex from a good and authentic source

Learn from reliable sources and investigate your sex attitudes. Investigate what your parents and upbringing taught you about sex. When you come across a detrimental belief, dispute it. If you require assistance, try speaking with doctors or a mental health professional.

These beliefs might have a negative impact on our sexual and mental health. To overcome these beliefs, we can make space for sexual learning and growth. We might strive for a more egalitarian sexual experience in which both partners feel loved, wanted, and respected. We can teach our sons and daughters that boys are sensitive, crave solid connections and that everyone is different. And last but not least, sex education should be a part of growing up.

Chapter 3
Why Sex Education Is Important?

In India, abortion-related illnesses claim the lives of 13 women every day, and the nation has the third-highest percentage of HIV patients. Every year, around 1.6 billion girls under 19 become pregnant. And still, sex education is considered taboo to talk about. If you are wondering what sex education is, it's simple, as the name suggests: the education of sex like other subjects in schools or on social platforms and gatherings. The goal of sex education is to help people understand issues related to sex, sexuality, and sexual health.

What Is Sex Education?

Sexual education is acquiring knowledge and understanding of the emotional, physical, and social aspects of sexuality. Sex education is giving information about body development, sex, sexuality, and relationships, as well as skill development, to assist young people in communicating about sex and making educated decisions about their sexual health. Sex education should be offered to pupils at all grade levels, with content tailored to their developmental stage and cultural background. Information on puberty and reproduction, abstinence, birth control, condoms, partnerships, avoidance of sexual violence, body image, gender identity, and sexual orientation should all be included.

It ought to be instructed by qualified teachers. Sex education should respect young people's access to complete and accurate information while also considering the best practices for preventing unwanted pregnancy and STDs. Sex education should emphasize that sexual development is a specific, natural aspect of human growth.

Objectives of Sex Education

Sex education aims to improve young people's attitudes regarding sexual and reproductive health behaviours and their understanding of men's and women's bodies. Knowing the differences and similarities between genders can help kids learn more about their bodies and how they change as they age. This approach will lay the groundwork for future growth in their acquaintance with their buddies or partners. Sex education instils a sense of responsibility in both others and oneself, and it is about accepting oneself and embracing one's body.

Importance of Sex Education

Sex Education makes things normal.

Adolescents do have difficulties as they reach puberty. People frequently misinterpret certain things as abnormal. Accept that your body is changing, whether physically or biologically. Sex education aids in the education and awareness of children. Whereas ignorance might cause individuals to despise their bodies or compare themselves to others their age, sex education can help you recognize what's expected.

Sex education makes people aware of hygiene.

As they say, "Your body is your temple," Take good care of your body. It becomes increasingly crucial to maintain a clean body as you age. Sex education provides vital information on how to maintain personal hygiene. Not all parents can teach their children these techniques, and it may be awkward to discuss these things with children. On the other hand, some parents must be aware of special safety measures when educating their kids about hygiene. Schools can hire qualified instructors with the necessary skills to assist students in learning more about their bodies and becoming more aware of them.

Sex Education makes awareness of safety.

Sex education protects kids by raising their understanding of how to protect themselves from sexually transmitted illnesses, sexual exploitation, sexual abuse, and other such dangers. Kids will be equipped to protect themselves from sexual exploitation. Furthermore, younger people become more vulnerable to several threats and risks as technology advances. Sex education makes students equipped to handle and overcome obstacles.

Sex Education eradicates gender discrimination.

Due to societal influence, young kids develop prejudiced attitudes against people of a specific gender. Sex education will empower students to advocate for gender equality and live a gender-equal lifestyle. It also teaches kids about their rights over their bodies and critical teachings such as the importance of permission in a sexual relationship, among other things. Sex education would help children learn about the LGBTQ population and the injustices they encounter. It teaches kids to treat everyone equally and respectfully, regardless of gender.

Sex Education provides reliable information.

Kids today have access to many types of information via the internet in our highly technological environment. Yet, the information people discover online can be different, and they may need to make better judgments due to the false information they are given. Sex education helps kids get the correct knowledge from specialists and apply the advice professionals provide daily.

Sex Education teaches Responsible behaviour

In addition to sex education teachings, kids will learn to act among people of any gender or age. When confronted with complex conditions, they will know what to do. They know how to respect others and open the door to discussing their problems with friends and family.

Sex Education helps to reduce Unplanned pregnancies.

Teens who engage in sexual activity without sufficient information are more likely to become pregnant unintentionally. Comprehensive sex education increases student confidence, improves judgment and conduct, and lowers danger. This reduces the frequency of unplanned pregnancies and enhances protection against infections and diseases spread through sexual contact.

Sex Education helps in building a healthy relationship.

Sex education assists a teen in differentiating between

good and bad relationships. Sex education is crucial in helping young people develop long-lasting, trusting relationships. It enables children to build healthy friendships while lowering their chances of entering unstable or toxic relationships. Furthermore, it encourages children to look for the appropriate resources and role models who can educate them on sex in a non-threatening setting.

Sex Education emphasizes the importance of consent.

Consent in a sexual relationship refers to both partners' agreement to engage in a given activity. This makes it simpler for individuals to stop participating in activities that they no longer find enjoyable. You will feel more confident about yourself as you learn about sex and how it affects your body. Sex education enables a person to make the best decision when confronted with sexual situations that are inappropriate for their age.

Sex Education tries to forbid risky situations.

Students who participate in sex education are forbidden from engaging in dangerous activities like sharing needles or having sex without protection, which can result in deadly illnesses. Sex education offers knowledge that protects against the dangers of unprotected sex. It also teaches children how to reject peer pressure and avoid circumstances in which they may be pressured to do anything that could endanger their health.

Sex Education make awareness of sexual assault.

Young people are taught what constitutes sexual violence through proper sexual education. Because they are unaware of the sexual exploitation they are subjected to, children are often reluctant to report it to their parents. Sexual violence is unacceptable, and children have the right to understand their bodies and seek help if abused.

Points to consider in Sex Education

- Sex education should be given to children based on age and developmental stage. The following are some points that must be followed:
- Proper use of body words and actions.
- Gender equality should be taught, and LGBTQ+ people should not be disparaged.
- Students are free to address any problem concerning sexuality in class.
- Students should avoid discussing other students' information or issues in class.
- Respect for one another.
- Students should refrain from discussing other students' information or issues in class.

Myths and Facts about Sex Education

The foundation of sex education is the belief that young people have a right to sexual education to make educated decisions about their sexuality and reproductive health. Despite proving the ability to assist youth in postponing the initiation of sexual activity, lowering the frequency and number of sexual assaults, and boosting condom and contraceptive usage, sex education is constantly under attack by society. It's time to end the discussion and dispel some more prevalent fallacies about sex education because so much false information is being spread about it.

Myth: Sex education disregards values

Fact: Excellent sex education promotes a rights-based perspective in which respect, acceptance, tolerance, equality, empathy, and reciprocity are intrinsically related to generally recognized human rights. Also, sex education allows young people to examine and clarify their values and those of their families and communities.

Myth: Sex education teaches the process of sex

Fact: Sex education offers skills and knowledge that are age- and developmentally appropriate to help young people put off sexual initiation and protect themselves when they do. Sexual education is intended to be developmentally and age-appropriate. The subjects presented differ by grade and are sequentially structured to develop young people's knowledge and skills as they mature. For instance, students learn about family structure, the correct names for body parts, and what to do if someone touches them improperly in kindergarten through second grade. Students in grades three to five studies about puberty and the physical changes that occur during this time. Also, they start to learn about HIV in an age-appropriate manner, including the fact that the virus cannot be spread by simple contact. Students in grades six through eight are taught about relationships, making decisions, being assertive, and developing their ability to withstand peer and social pressure. In later grades, they learn about sexually transmitted diseases, pregnancy, and safety precautions.

Myth: Sex education encourages sex

Fact: Although scientifically incorrect, many individuals think like that, and the reality is that sexual and reproductive health education does not promote more sexual activity. Instead, those with access to thorough sex education feel more confident about their sexuality, postpone sexual activity, and use contraception more frequently.

Myth: Sex education should be taught by parents only

Fact: The first educators in a child's life are their parents and legal guardians. They educate the views and values, either explicitly or through example. They exchange information and respond to questions. During many years of regular contact, they scaffold the teaching of challenging concepts. Not every parent feels prepared to discuss sensitive issues such as relationships and sexuality. Most young people want informed and comfortable adults and educators to teach them about sexuality, health, and relationships. Young people have many questions and want to learn, so providing them with many opportunities is beneficial! Parents and schools can work together to achieve this goal.

Myth: Sex education is not important as other subjects

Fact: Sex education is just as vital as any other subject. Sex education focuses on developing the knowledge and skills to live healthy lives, have healthy relationships, and thrive. Having the knowledge and skills necessary to make healthy decisions, take care of your body, and treat others and yourself with respect is what sex-ed means when done correctly. As a society, this entails addressing significant concerns such as increased STI rates, discrimination, and gender-based violence. Obtaining such education has the potential to transform our lives profoundly.

When you say the word sex in front of a group of people, or worse, in front of your parents, you may feel embarrassed and awkward. Sex has long been associated with ugliness, filth, and immortality. One of the foundations of society is human sexuality, although it has long been considered impure. However, some families and schools frequently refuse to explain or warn their minors about this, which causes misunderstandings about sexuality and sexual health in children and teenagers. Why do we feel uncomfortable talking about sex, or being considered taboo? Let's know why talking about sex is taboo in the family, and parents don't teach kids about sexuality.

Talking about sex will encourage kids to engage more in it

Some parents fear that by discussing their bodies and sexuality openly with their kids, they either endorse or allow promiscuous conduct. However, the truth is that most sexually active teenagers are usually the least informed. Generally, silence and ignorance, rather than open dialogue, lead to poor decisions. The more solid sexual information children receive from their parents, the better equipped they are to make moral and mature decisions. According to some research, parents who talk to their children about sex postpone their children's sexual involvement because they fulfill their children's curiosity, often leading to experimenting.

Parents felt embarrassed to talk about sex

The simple fact is that many parents find it

embarrassing to talk about these topics with their kids. The most challenging and delicate subject parents must discuss with their kids is sexuality, and most parents would be too afraid even to consider having such a conversation. I remember one incident where a 15-year-old girl asked her mother about her body changes, and she put a book on her bed and avoided the discussion. The mother's embarrassment fostered the daughter's discomfort and contributed to the daughter's increasing notion that sex was an unmentionable human sorrow.

Negative Conditioning of Parents

Parents' shame results from their own sexual inadequacies and unresolved limiting beliefs. Parents often lack the necessary self-awareness even to acknowledge that they may have some problems. Many parents believe they don't need to teach their children about sex because their parents never did. Parents today do not have the luxury of avoiding this critical topic. For today's youth, this is a "must-have" information and comprehension to teach with purely positive light and truth; parents must become conscious of and deal with their own unfavorable attitudes and ideas.

Children are also embarrassed to talk with their parents

Parents are ashamed, and many youngsters are mortified by sex talk. This happens when parents miss the opportunity to teach their kids about sex while they are still "blank slates" and before they have formed negative associations with the subject. It's simpler to teach and uphold the idea that sex is precious and sacred - not disgusting – if parents start enlightening their kids at a young age.

Weak parent-child relationship

When parents struggle to connect with their children, it can be incredibly challenging to bring up such a sensitive and complex issue as sex. The discussion of sex is much more Taboo when a parent and child have problems. Before having intimate chats, parents may need to invest time and effort in mending the bond. To prevent their kids from needing to find fake love and fulfillment, parents can do a lot to meet their kids' emotional needs and build a stronger bond with them.

Lack of Sex education

Sex is Taboo in many households because many parents don't know what to say about it, let alone when or how to mention it. Parents may feel uneasy about their understanding if they weren't properly educated about sex as children and haven't tried to study it. Thinking about the questions today's teenagers might ask can be daunting! Some parents might believe it's too late now that their kids are grown up or that they are too young for such a conversation. Some may even think they don't need to learn because they'll figure it out once married! Isn't sex essential and natural? What is there to know? This way of thinking reveals a lack of knowledge about the female sexual response and the interplay between emotional, spiritual, and physical intimacy.

How to break this Taboo?

The only way to break this Taboo is to talk about it. Even though discussing sex can be one of the most challenging, it is also one of the most crucial. To have good relationships and engage in safe sex, we must talk frankly and honestly about sex. Many people find it awkward to talk about sex, but avoiding the subject can hinder communication, cause misunderstandings in

relationships, and even put people at risk for STIs.

How to Start Conversation:

Many people find it challenging to initiate a sex talk, mainly if they aren't used to it. Here are some suggestions about how to start a conversation:

- Choose a relaxing environment, and pick a location that makes you feel at ease and home.
- Choose the right time and a quiet period to avoid interruptions or other disturbances.
- Keep an open-ended conversation; if talking with kids, ask, "What do they want to ask? And what are their thoughts about?" and clarify their doubts and explain. And When talking with your partner, converse about a healthy sexual relationship.
- Be mindful of the other person's comfort zone and boundaries. If they feel uncomfortable discussing it, respect their freedom to refuse or shift the topic.
- Listen and pay attention to what the other person is saying and be open to diverse points of view.

Why it's important to talk about sex

It's crucial to discuss sex since it enables us to comprehend our partner's needs, expectations, and boundaries. This can help us better understand our partner's needs and preferences, which can help us develop closeness, trust, and respect in our relationship. Candid discussions about sex can also assist us in identifying potential dangers, ensuring that we are engaging in safe sex and abstaining from dangerous habits. Some of the important causes are described further down.

- Maintaining good sexual health is among the most crucial justifications for discussing sex. People can better understand the potential risks of sexual activity and be equipped to take protective measures by having open and honest conversations about sex. The risk of sexually transmitted infections (STIs) can be decreased by encouraging people to engage in safe sexual behavior. People can better understand their own bodies and their own sexual needs and desires by having sex and by talking about it. This can assist in guaranteeing that sexual encounters are pleasurable and consenting. It may be challenging for some people to talk about their sexual health, and they may be medical professionals. In these situations, it's critical to remember that discussing sex is a sign of strength, not weakness.
- Speaking openly about sex is crucial for educating others about healthy boundaries, consent, and sexual relationships. Young people, frequently exposed to false or outdated information from peers or the media, should pay particular attention to this. People can better understand what kinds of sexual behavior are healthy and acceptable by having open and honest conversations about sex. This can ensure that individuals can make educated decisions regarding their sexual conduct and the legal and social repercussions of participating in particular behaviors.
- It is also necessary to discuss sex to confront antiquated

attitudes and beliefs. People, for example, can assist in removing the stigma surrounding topics such as LGBTQ+ partnerships, sex work, and another sexual expressions by discussing sex in a positive, respectful manner.

- Having sex-related conversations can also help with mental wellness. Many people experience emotions of shame or embarrassment over their sexual aspirations or behaviors, which can result in feelings of guilt, anxiety, and low self-esteem. People might feel more at ease with themselves and their sexuality by having non-judgmental conversations about sex. This can assist in alleviating feelings of shame and fear, making it easier to discuss sexual concerns with partners or healthcare providers.
- Speaking about sex can assist in alleviating the pressure to conform to specific sexual norms or expectations. Individuals may be concerned that their sexual preferences or behaviors are "weird" or "strange." Still, by discussing sex freely, they might discover no "correct" way to express their sexuality.

Conclusion

Society-structured cultural norms and values hold that sex should never be publicly discussed. Because it is a profoundly private act in which two people express compassion, many cultures do not allow open conversations or depictions of such events. The main reason that schools and parents frequently fail to provide sex education and adults don't openly discuss their sexual health or preferences is because of society's projection that talking about sex is such a repulsive activity.

Kids who form healthier opinions about their bodies, their interactions with others, and their interactions with people at home and abroad will grow up to be capable individuals who can handle any scenario. To make informed judgments, young people require reliable information from an adult they can trust, and instructors can ensure that they deliver accurate information to their students. Accurate information from reputable people can have a long-term favorable impact on their sexual health. The inclusion of sex education in school curricula can help young people develop positive attitudes and actions that can be reinforced throughout their lives in a variety of ways. **"Don't consider sex talk taboo; talk freely and confidently."**

Chapter 4
Kamasutra

In India, the word "sex" is considered taboo, yet our population is still expanding. Most Indians believe it is improper to teach kids about Sex at home or in school. We continue to have children in a nation where the family, the state, and other institutions have suppressed the topic and surpassed China in population.

However, we must remember that three basic needs stand out: food, water, and reproduction. While food and water are crucial for an individual's existence, reproduction is essential for the survival of society. Most individuals find the process enjoyable, but it transcends mere enjoyment in other cultures. It is respected as art and occasionally even revered as a religious ideal. Some refer to it as Sex, while others refer to it as a way of life. This is when the Kama Sutra enters the picture.

What is Kamasutra

The "Kama Sutra" was composed in India between AD 320 and 550, during the Gupta Golden Period, by a religious scholar and philosopher named Vatsyayana. The book is technically religious literature because it is based on

Hinduism. According to Hinduism, everyone must fulfill the four fundamentals of life:

Dharma (Duty): Dharma covers one's religious obligations, moral obligations, and obligations to uphold good conduct and ethical principles. It also includes actions that support societal order.

Artha (Purpose): Artha combines money, a successful profession, and a job that allows you to earn a livelihood and achieve financial stability and economic prosperity. In Hinduism, people must adequately pursue artha.

Kama (Desire): It denotes, with or without sexual overtones, affection, love, the pleasure of the senses, passion, emotions, and aesthetic enjoyment of life.

Moksha (Self-Actualization): Moksha refers to liberation, self-awareness, self-realization, and freedom in this life.

The Kamasutra served as a manual dealing with the purpose of desire, lust, and the philosophy of love. Sex and sexuality were essential aspects of Indian society in ancient India. Particularly among the elite classes, polygamy and polyamory were widespread. Sex was viewed as a marital obligation for the wife and the husband. Despite being private, both partners were supposed to enjoy themselves throughout the deed.

Facts about Kamasutra

- Many people think of Kamasutra as Erotica; however, only one chapter out of seven discusses sexuality. Kamasutra covers much more ground than we might think. This book gives romance guidance, marriage advice, and even having an affair. However, having an affair doesn't mean committing adultery; it is just a gentle reminder for husbands to take care of their spouses.

- The Kama Sutra is intended to be a manual to help both sexual partners enjoy themselves most naturally. It's not intended to be a list of erotic sexual positions you can check off. Sex isn't meant to be osteopathic agony; the postures are presented as suggestions rather than prescriptions. The goal is always enjoyable, not practicing a position for months.
- Understanding how to draw the appropriate kind of a person into your life is crucial to finding a permanent partner. In addition to the first physical appeal, you must have compatible personalities. The Kama Sutra contains two chapters devoted to instruction on increasing physical attraction with possible spouses and, if that attraction has been established, how to ignite sexual power.
- Only five chapters are devoted to the procedures and theories involved in finding a bride, while further chapters discuss the interaction with a wife once the marriage has been consummated. Traditional wisdom deals with making a girl feel comfortable around you and keeping her as yours forever. This advice applies even in contemporary society, where dating is considerably more casual, and matrimonial websites can introduce and lessen the initial discomfort between a possible pair.

Attributes of Kamasutra

- The Kamasutra is the result of a civilization that sought to comprehend human life in all its manifestations. The pursuit of pleasure and happiness, including sexual pleasure, was investigated in the Upanishads, ancient Indian philosophical literature.
- Kamasutra explains the unity of all human attributes. The mind and the physical body are not different entities, nor are sentiments and emotions; they are the life force when they are all together. The five elements and the material and spiritual worlds are not two distinct realms, just as the human species is not separate from nature. Being forms of energy, the physical and material are likewise spiritual and deserve equal reverence. The human body, like the soul, is heavenly.
- Kamasutra's goal is to demonstrate how paradoxes should be used to understand and experience life because paradoxes are a part of human existence. All the factors that produce sexual pleasure and satisfaction are found outside of sexuality, the sexual pleasure paradox. Self-interest is paradoxical in that one can only advance their own interests by advancing those of others. In other words, one's joy and happiness are dependent on the pleasure and satisfaction of others. The paradox of the self is that it cannot exist without the other. Also, perhaps most importantly, there is the paradox of limits, which is the idea that one can only become aware of their boundaries by going beyond them.
- According to Kamasutra, everything that happens in

human life depends on the "right place," "suitable time," and "appropriate person." These three must be constantly combined to understand the purpose and beauty of life and relationships.

- According to the Kamasutra, the body is as sacred as the soul, and sexuality is as revered as the spiritual in all its tangible manifestations. They flow into one other like energy to create life's joy. Separating them based on the utterly erroneous belief that one is coarse and the other refined, one at a lower and one at a higher level of consciousness, is a form of self-violence from the outset since it is an attack on human worth. In short, joy cannot exist apart from reverence.
- In the first few pages of Kamasutra, Vatsyayana explained that eroticism permeates sexuality such that it can be felt, not simply sensed, for a short time. A wholesome relationship between a man and a woman demands, first and foremost, a healthy relationship with one's self, in which no one human quality is torn from the others and then becomes the only basis of one's life. Even in its own terms, developing a much broader range of sensibilities, such as those for music, dance, poetry, and literature, would be necessary for the art of making love. And it is what the Kamasutra's author, Vatsyayana, implies in the first few pages.

The Kama Sutra is more than you might believe; it's a helpful guide for learning to lead a happy life. Desire, sexual pleasure, and emotional contentment are listed as appropriate life goals in the Kama Sutra. Its numerous chapters include topics such as finding a mate, flirting, retaining adequate power in married life, social engagement training, and, as we all know, some advice and thoughts regarding sexual positions. Sex is the art of creating love, physical pleasure, and happiness, and there are numerous lessons to be learned from Kamasutra.

Without passing judgment on morality, ancient literature outlines numerous forms of sexual pleasure available to men and women. Kamasutra was written about 1,500 years ago: the author, Vatsyayana, made it clear that his knowledge was common and that he had drawn on various authors and sources to put it together.

While Lodhi kings governed Delhi in the 15th century, a sex manual called Ananga Ranga was written. Its goal differed: teaching men how to appease their spouses so they would remain devoted to their marriages. However, Ananga Ranga, like Kamashastra, discusses alchemical aphrodisiacs for greater masculinity and the role astrology might play in attracting love and sparking passion. Though sex education has been incorporated into our culture for a long time, modern society is not ready to add sex education to school or college curricula and make us feel ashamed of having sexual desire. As we discussed the importance of healthy Sex and myths related to it in our previous chapter, lovemaking is not limited to the act of having Sex. There are more layers to it that we will discuss in the next chapter.

Chapter 5
Foreplay

Every couple knows that a strong marriage depends on regular, intense sexual connection. Several people have realized this due to rich, fulfilling personal experiences, and others have discovered the lesson by accident, as their relationships suffer because of a lack of Sex. However, many people in both categories are unaware that Sex is more than sexual activity.

Our culture attempts to convince us that Sex is most effective when kept as separate from the rest of our daily experience as possible using various subtle and not-so-subtle means, like movies, television, and steamy literature. On the other hand, our Scripture takes a very opposite stance. According to Kamasutra, Sex is all about understanding the other person, in and out, and comprehensive understanding that embraces complete mutuality and total sharing in all aspects of life. If we say meaningful Sex is like baking a multilayer cake, you must work on each layer to bake a perfect and satisfying cake. Like cake, Sex also has many layers before reaching the end point of sexual intercourse. Let's talk about the first layer of Sex, "foreplay."

In Sex, Foreplay is considered the ideal preparatory action, preparing the body for distinct pleasures. Experts claim that before sex starts, two people engage in enticing behaviors such as hugging, kissing, touching, or stripping. The initial sexual contact before a sexual encounter is referred to as Foreplay. Although it is an essential element of the sexual experience, Foreplay is often undervalued.

Importance of Foreplay

The act of Foreplay is crucial because it fosters sexual arousal, strengthens romantic bonds, and encourages the idea of sharing emotions between the two bodies.

Amid Foreplay, you and your partner will exist in a world of just the two of you, giving and receiving a broad spectrum of feelings without giving it a second thought. Hugging, kissing, and other touching gestures will encourage deep bodily joy. In a nutshell, Foreplay underpins the sense of emotion and excitement. Though there are various benefits to Foreplay, let's check its importance from biological and psychological perspectives.

Importance of Foreplay in Biological Perspective

From a biological standpoint, women must engage in Foreplay. The arousal increases during premarital contact, resulting in a clitoris erection. Similar to how the penis works, the clitoris also does. To experience an orgasm, the clitoris must be erected due to the blood flow there. Moreover, Foreplay causes vaginal moisture, facilitating painless and more effortless subsequent penetration for both the man and the woman. The lack of vaginal moisture makes sexual contact unpleasant and can occasionally result in minor bleeding. And remember, Foreplay is essential for both men and women.

Importance of Foreplay in Psychological Perspective

Foreplay reduces vulnerability and fosters a sense of security. According to reports, the absence of Foreplay leaves many people feeling ignored and robbed of the emotional security they require. It improves a couple's bond outside of the bedroom. Foreplay is key for long-term partnerships since it enhances sentiments of connection. Foreplay is also vital in making the partner feel you are paying attention to and caring about them. It is critical in instilling psychological safety and emotional well-being.

In a nutshell, Foreplay provides a way to enjoy sexual pleasure, focusing on enjoying the process rather than focusing on the end goal. We know that Foreplay can be confusing for many as various myths relate to it, and let us make it easy for you to understand by debunking these myths.

Myth #1 Sex should be effortless, and Foreplay is a waste of time

Fact: Foreplay not only makes Sex better but also enhances your relationship with your partner outside the bedroom by improving emotional intimacy.

Myth #2 Foreplay must start only in bed before Sex

Fact: If a woman can see that a man has a sensitive side in addition to a hot and passionate one, she will feel more connected to him and more prepared for a fantastic sex session. This indicates that Foreplay doesn't always need to come before a sexual act. It can include sensual eye contact while making supper or anything else that makes your lover feel appreciated.

Myth #3 Oral Sex and Foreplay are synonyms for each other

Fact: It's absolutely a myth because Foreplay doesn't need to involve genitals to make your partner turn on. It's all about communicating with each other and sharing what they like and doesn't like. In other words, Foreplay is all about creating small beautiful moments with each other.

Myth #4 Foreplay is Time-Restricted

Fact: Some people view Foreplay as merely an activity they must complete to meet a minimum time requirement that leads to sexual intercourse. However, there is no set duration for Foreplay; nonetheless, it comprises a steady rise in sexual desire and tension. Foreplay timing depends on mood, energy level, and surroundings.

Myth #5 Foreplay always leads to Sex

Fact: Not always. Foreplay is entertaining on its own and has not required Sex to follow. Factors like our emotions can impact arousal. Don't feel obligated to have Sex if you're not interested. Even after Foreplay, you don't owe somebody sex.

Now that you understand why Foreplay is essential, let's learn more about it:

How do you decide what to do or what you don't like about what your partner is doing?

Regarding Foreplay, there are no specific dos and don'ts. It would help to learn about your partner's likes and dislikes on the go. Pay attention to the cues, and make each other feel at ease. Foreplay can sometimes be awkward, and having Sex can make us all feel exposed, especially if we're trying something new or are with a new partner. So, communication is the key; communicate with each other and say frankly, "This doesn't feel right to me; let's try other things."

Intimacy and Foreplay Tips

Kamasutra has a unique quality, and it has countless hints and tips up its sleeve. The ancient Vedic Scripture contains in-depth advice on Sex, pleasure, and desire that both men and women may use to enhance their sex lives. It is not limited to sexual intercourse but also extends beyond basic Sex. You're seeking Foreplay, which can be as delightful and passionate as possible. As a result, here are some Kamasutra foreplay suggestions to help you increase your bedroom time!

Embrace your partner

To begin with, it is not simply hugging but also touching your partner's whole body. Intimate contact will start to rekindle the flame and cause pleasure to spread between the partners. This process naturally awakened the lengthy touching period, and an embrace like this fosters a love relationship between you and your spouse.

Importance of Kiss

Do not hurry into it. Take your time and carefully explore your partner's lips. It becomes more erogenous as it becomes slower and more sensual. Start by lightly touching their lips, then gradually turn up the heat. If you intend to have Sex, this is the finest technique to turn on your partner.

Scratching and Biting

After kissing, you can begin raking your partner's body with your nails since it creates a raw, alluring, and steamy feeling. Ladies enjoy scratching their partners' bodies and hanging tight when things get passionate and wild!

If done delicately, biting can be highly sexually exciting. It can be erotic for you and your lover because biting on the sensory zones can significantly improve sexual stimulation. It also correlates with the mechanics of domination in bed.

For relationships that are meant to last, foreplay is important. Maintaining a connection and intimacy with our partners is important when life gets in the way - our kids, our work, our stress, finances, whatever it is - and foreplay helps to do that.

Intimacy can be maintained via foreplay; both mental and physical intimacy. Foreplay can not only increase sex for you and your partner (regardless of your gender), but it can also strengthen your bond outside of the bedroom. Increasing foreplay isn't the only method to have successful sex, but for most individuals, it's significant overall. The most important factor in a successful relationship is that both partners are sexually pleased. So long as you're making sure that's rewarding for you and your spouse, it's okay if your relationship lives on the occasional quickies. So, foreplay is important not only for healthy sex life, also for physical and mental health. The feeling of being loved is irreplaceable.

Chapter 6

Roleplay Or Safeplay?

Role Play

Marrying your true love and falling in love with them daily is fantastic. But, even the healthiest unions are not immune from stale periods. The secret might be getting into roleplaying to get your sex life moving and shaking once more.

Roleplaying is a game of make-believe in which you can become whatever you want and associate with anybody. It's unnecessary to spend a fortune on a hotel room or wear out your budget on outrageous outfits to roleplay. The only thing you have to do is choose a scene or fantasy that you like, and then try to live it out.

What is Role Play

Consenting partners will pretend to be various characters in a made-up story while having sex, known as "sexual role play". To guarantee permission, partners generally discuss fantasy roleplaying scenarios beforehand. A roleplaying session might be straightforward or intricate, involving dressing up, traveling to a fantastical setting, invoking a backstory from a favorite film or television program, and more.

You have the chance to, through Roleplay, "make routine in a long-term relationship more exciting. It facilitates reaching a "greater level of intimacy" as a result of a willingness on the part of both partners to divulge more personal information. Roleplaying provides a couple with a secure environment to examine their relationship and discover a new side of themselves. Roleplaying can help you and your partner communicate better while increasing arousal in your relationship. The deeper the emotional connection and bonding, the more you may discuss your desires and let yourself be exposed by acting out a scene.

Benefits of Roleplay

A good marriage requires intimacy and sex in addition to the other essentials of love, kindness, respect, and generosity that make up a happy and healthy partnership. To spice up their marriages, couples turn to fantasy and roleplaying. There are many advantages to roleplaying for a beautiful and healthy married life.

Safe Place for Relationship

Roleplaying allows a safe place for couples and their fantasies with the security of long-term relationships. Many people are concerned that their urge to roleplay will make them look foolish, yet this couldn't be further from the truth. Roleplaying is a private method to discover each other's dreams and let your guard down with your partner.

Role Play builds trust

Investigating role play in the bedroom has several

advantages, including that "playing out a fantasy typically takes place when a person feels extremely safe and secure in a relationship. Roleplaying is acting out your own or a partner's desires. "Roleplaying can indicate how safe you feel with your partner for sex, both physically and emotionally." Trust, of course, works both ways. Always be honest with your spouse if they bring up a fantasy, just as you would want them to create a secure and private space for you to explore yours.

Role play helps in healing

Many people are unaware of this, but roleplaying can be a highly healing activity for the couple and the individuals involved. It's easy to become mired in everyday routines, stalled at work, etc., and it is crucial to change things up because of this occasionally. Roleplaying enables sexual partners to have fun, escape reality, and ultimately let go. It could be therapeutic in specific ways for both parties.

Roleplay helps to know about your partner

Although it's occasionally our propensity to think we completely understand our partners, the likelihood is that we don't. This doesn't imply that they are keeping something from you or doing something evil; instead, it just means that there is always more to discover about a person, and roleplaying could be a terrific way to do so.

Roleplay rekindles the spark

Feeling pumped up and eager for intimacy can be challenging after spending much time together. Nevertheless, it is sad that many relationships sometimes become uninteresting as years of marriage luster when couples settle like old flour in a jar and have the same old routine. No doubt, communication, respect, and love are the cornerstones of a successful marriage, but will these factors be enough to keep the flame burning? Roleplaying can revive the passion and provide a special spark to long-term relationships. Furthermore, it also requires much intimacy. Finding and openly expressing each other's darkest dreams and playing them out with your partners helps deepen the mate bond. Being exploratory can help a couple develop their relationship and become more intimate.

Roleplay improves the communication

You will grow closer to your lover if you share your deepest wishes and fantasies. Communication between the two of you will become more straightforward as they learn to comprehend some of your underlying goals and requirements. Roleplaying can help you express what you want from your partner openly and honestly since it will help you understand your wishes.

Roleplaying increases your partner's level of commitment to the relation

A healthy sex life invariably reduces a spouse's urge to wander, even if you shouldn't ever feel compelled to do something you aren't entirely comfortable with only to please your partner. Why would people travel elsewhere if they could get everything in one place?

Roleplay is the safest way to make your fantasy true

You don't have to be concerned about affairs, STDs, or broken feelings. You play a distinctive role while appreciating each other's roles in a secure environment. The most excellent part is that you envision yourself in a story with a stranger, but behind that stranger is your loved one, and you are free from guilt or wrongdoing.

Roleplaying facilitates self-discovery

Even while having sex is undoubtedly a two-person activity, there are instances when it can reveal more about you than anybody else. You may discover facts about yourself that you were unaware of by investigating your deepest passions.

How to Initiate Roleplay

Determine your goals

Addressing your desires with your spouse can be scary, mainly if you've never discussed roleplaying. Consider what you hope to gain from your first roleplaying experience as you prepare for that first dialogue. Do you wish to do something new in front of others, such as meeting a stranger in a bar? Do you want to stage a full-fledged, period-piece recreation in your house in costume? Do you want to focus on a "business partner" narrative that is more formal and businesslike? In any case, sort through all the familiar fantasy tales in your thoughts and decide which one feels the most believable and attractive.

Discuss or talk to your partner

Of course, you'll want to discuss this with your spouse beforehand, and you should agree on your approaches and the necessary consent. Because role play is rather complicated and would require a specific level of dedication from both parties, it feels vital to have an initial talk. But it is optional for you to present a wholly developed action plan. Instead, start slowly. You may find out if your partner has any recurring fantasies. Determine the nature of their specific roleplay ideals. Finally, see if you can combine or attempt each independently to guarantee that everyone feels heard.

Develop a plan together

Discuss your game plan with your partner for the more important roleplaying exercise. No, you don't have to plan out the entire evening. Yet, you must agree on a few crucial points to fully assume the role and immerse yourself in the experience. What will you be wearing? Do you use accents? Do you decorate your place appropriately? Regardless of your favorite method, you must work together to complete this role play, so talk through your expectations beforehand.

Begin by using simple props

A full-on theatrical experience may sound fun to some of us, but for others, it may have more "drama club" than "sex appeal" appeal. Most experts advise starting slowly to avoid experiencing this as a high school play. We're not suggesting you can't advance on this front by any means. Furthermore, overdoing your costume predicament can prevent you from immersing yourself in your selected narrative. We advise beginning simple and easing into more significant roleplay scenarios.

Have fun without fear

This may seem silly at first. That is true, after all. In addition, it allows you to explore new ground with your spouse while giving in to some of your most intense and long-standing dreams. Hence, remember that it's okay to chuckle through a few steps here. It means you two are having fun together and might need to take your time, but it doesn't mean you can't get into character.

This may seem like putting yourself out there, but remember that this is your partner. If you can't be honest with them, you could have deeper issues that roleplaying can't necessarily help. Remember that this is a collaborative effort. Don't be offended if your spouse hesitates to participate in the conversation; let them be. Accept that you will take tiny steps as long as you enjoy the direction.

Tips to consider before Roleplay

Review the following tips and principles before engaging in a hot scenario with your partner:

Talk and list down your sexual desires: Discuss scenarios and roles you'd like to try before attempting a scene with your partner. Choose the finest sex situation for both of you that simulates an exciting and entertaining dynamic.

Make your bedroom a judgment-free zone: You need to discuss your thoughts and desires without fear of being judged to have truly fantastic sex. Agree with your partner before roleplaying that you won't ever mock each other's sexual performance, fantasies, or decisions—and that you will keep your sex life secret. Don't discuss graphic details with anyone, not even your closest friend. Sex is fragile, and to thoroughly explore it freely, we must be confident that our tendencies will not be revealed to others. You will feel more at ease leaning into your kinky sides after you have that assurance out of the way.

Understand that fantasy is not always politically and morally correct: Our desires in bed frequently conflict with our ideologies and how we view ourselves. Roleplaying fantasies conflict with how people conduct themselves in public. Since these desires are so utterly at odds with what we desire and experience in our daily lives, it can be challenging to embrace them as pieces of who we are. Yet, toying with power in bed is different from desiring the scenario to happen; these wants only exist on one level, and we need to be willing to accept that compartmentalization. As long as it's mutually agreed upon, the bedroom should be a space where we can play with power, submission, role reversal, danger, and even degradation. And we must do it without feeling embarrassed or judged by ourselves or our relationships.

Set Limits: Establishing boundaries before you become a character is crucial because you might say or do exciting and amusing things in the roleplaying environment but inappropriate things elsewhere. You may have agreed to act out a fantasy, but that doesn't mean you have consented to any course it may take. Moreover, consent may lapse. It would help if you had a safety phrase during roleplaying because sometimes we agree to things, but they don't feel good when we perform them.

Suspend your disbelief: When roleplaying, people frequently feel foolish and ridiculous. To get to the pleasurable stuff, you must overcome your self-judgment. Try it out by setting a time limit on how long you'll commit to acting in character; the longer the period, the less awkward you'll feel. But, the most crucial commitment during roleplaying is to refrain from judging yourself or your partner. It's the key to unlocking the numerous sexy characters within you both.

Spent time after sex: After the roleplaying is finished, talk about the experience with your spouse while cuddling after a sexual encounter. Give your thoughts on what you enjoyed and disliked about the event and what you'd like to do differently next time.

How Often Should Roleplay

Roleplaying is beneficial when it can be tried out sometimes. To renew the excitement during sex, once every few weeks is a decent quantity. Nevertheless, if you have too much of it, you and your partner start to rely on having separate personalities when having sex. This can play on your subconscious mind and make you both crave a different, fabricated version of each other. As a result, you and your lover can engage in roleplaying during sex on occasion but don't make it a routine.

Safe Play the Role Play

Political correctness need not apply to your fantasy, and social acceptability is not required. It is neither uncommon nor pathological to have fantasies considered examples of "man's inhumanity to man." Before beginning this activity, you should negotiate with all persons involved and obtain their approval while being honest about your intentions. While thinking of roleplaying, negotiation, boundaries, and consent are crucial. Without them, your chances of making mistakes that ruin fun or, worse yet, cause emotional havoc increase. If expectations are unclear and no one is on the same page, even a lighthearted, enjoyable moment might go awry.

Consider and prepare for the situation while considering your partner's motives, desires, likes and dislikes, requirements, and preferences. The sky is the limit, but you and your companion must travel on the same page. The negotiation process, which involves establishing parameters for what is and is not acceptable, developing the intended scenario, and determining how long the scene will last, can appear tedious and like a huge chore.

Establishing boundaries is essential regardless of the roles you are contemplating. You've got to know where the edges of things are, whether you're the passive hostage, the forceful ravisher, or the more innocent self. Some people are great at improvising and just winging it, while others must know precisely what is around every corner to feel secure. Make sure you understand your boundaries, as well as the boundaries of your spouse.

An effective negotiating tactic is to share detailed and passionate fantasies. Many people appreciate hearing an excellent bawdy story, which might be the key to unlocking your secret garden. While being exposed in this way can be frightening, it significantly boosts your chances of your fantasy becoming a reality. Just safe play the roleplaying game to maintain your healthy and happy relationship!

Chapter 7 If It's Normal Why Is It A Taboo?

Taboos operate on the tenet of restricting or forbidding a person or group from engaging in a particular behavior by designating it as "unacceptable." But what is so surprising is taboos are subject to change. Earlier, we discussed how sex has to be normalised and why sex education is important. However, still, a majority portion of the adult society who have enough knowledge and have experienced sex still have a biased take on the basis of gender. The point of discussion here is not about if sex is normal, then why it is taboo; the motive of discussion in this chapter is why it is normal for some & why it is taboo for some.

Society grows to perceive sex: as a mystery. Within familial systems, by forcibly enforced caste limits, and by sexual censorship in the media, sexuality is a highly regulated area of life. The actual patterns of sexual behavior may not match the societal ideal. For instance, in the more conservative parts of the world, males aspire to be self-assured, powerful, honorable, and brave machos. Machos should be blatantly macho and sexually active; they will probably have one or more mistresses, a wife, and numerous children. Males are commonly thought to be naturally unfaithful. Contrarily, women are supposed to be submissive to their husbands' desires and engage in a sexual activity solely with them during the marriage. They must be chaste like the Virgin Mary.

Most parents struggle with having "the conversation" with their kids. As a result, they often forget that there are plenty of resources available for kids to learn about their bodies, which are frequently unreliable. Children who grow up in such a toxic environment learn to hide their curiosity from their parents. Nonetheless, there are differences between how teenage guys and girls display their sexuality. Males are more likely than girls to be socially accepted for having sexual experiences or learning about them since society has permitted boys to be overtly sexual creatures and glorify it by saying, "Men will be Men!"

The Truth of Female Sexuality in Patriarchal Society

Most millennial women are fed a balanced diet of things not to do, things not to know, things that aren't okay, and things others will say. As a result, we are taught to hide things from ourselves, not explore our own bodies or push sexual boundaries, to be likeable, and to keep our opinions to ourselves, among other things. Despite being compelled to follow a certain masculine stereotype, boys can talk openly about their sexuality, whereas girls are much less likely to do so because of the guilt they have been raised with. As a result, a widespread (and incorrect) perception develops that girls are the ones wanted rather than the ones wanting and devoid of sexual desire.

This misunderstanding stems from a fundamentally patriarchal worldview based on power relations in which the man is the provider, and the woman is the receiver. The subject-object status of a man and woman must remain in place for a patriarchal society to flourish. When a woman exhibits desire, it immediately exposes her place as a submissive object. Society does all in its power to quell it, frequently donning the guise of moral or religious ideas.

Sexual Myths Related to Female Sexuality

Women do not do masturbation

We all have generally believed this throughout life. This misconception is based on the assumption that women do not have separate desires from men. Second, it is "immoral" for a woman to touch herself. Third, only men can satisfy women, and they should do so. Masturbation helps a woman feel more in control of her body and understand what brings her the greatest pleasure.

Porn is not for women

There is little doubt that male audiences are the target audience for mainstream porn. This exemplifies that pornographers never needed to create "sex-positive" pornography, propagating the unequal power dynamics in cissexual relationships and presuming that women are non-desirous beings. However, a female porn director "Erika Lust" believes that both partners are sexually liberated equals.

A woman's Clitoris is an extraneous portion of her anatomy

In the female anatomy, Clitoris is in charge of "pleasure" and "feeling". The shockingly high number of FGM instances and the latest news story about Farida Bano's case illustrate how female desire has been suppressed for over a decade. Although Bano's mutilation took place in India, where a religious cult still holds that "the removal of the clitoris is the will of God," most mutilations still occur in Africa. Sadly, the government refuses to declare female circumcision a crime since it has a strong religious foundation, even though it is unquestionably a violation of human rights.

This is a foolish notion! While vaginal intercourse is delightful, researchers believe that over 70–80% of women have orgasms predominantly through clitoral stimulation. In truth, penetration does not generate orgasm; stimulation of the clitoris is the primary source of orgasm.

It is 'immoral' for a woman to lose her virginity before the marriage

Men don't have exact expectations regarding virginity; thus, they are free to engage in as many sexual experiences as they like before marriage without fear of social stigma. However, if a man stays a virgin for a long time, a patriarchal system frequently labels him as "unmanly" or looks down on him. The situation for women is entirely different, and there are no logical justifications for the same. Before getting married, women are supposed to be chaste." Even a sexual assault would cause a woman to lose her virginity, making her "unchaste" and letting their husbands do anything they want with their bodies because they are their husbands. The fact that marital rape is still not regarded as a crime in India.

Women's sexuality is till they reproduce

Women's sexuality is always directly proportional to their ability to bear children. There is a myth that menopause is the end of a woman's sexuality since she loses the ability to reproduce. However, a live example of Madonna breaks every stereotype and proves that age and the biological clock don't define women's sexuality.

Women are less interested in sex than males

Almost everyone has heard or assumed something similar to this prevalent myth. Let's be clear: This is stupid, based only on assumptions, and judgmental! The idea that women are less interested in initiating or desiring sex than men is untrue. According to studies, women crave sex just as much as men, but they tend to hold back because they are worried about being labeled "sluts". Women tend to be comparatively less open about their wants because of society's backward attitude toward female sexuality. Because they have a high sexual desire, some women even wonder whether there is something wrong with them due to this. To be clear, there is nothing wrong with having a sex drive.

Women are less sexually adventurous than men

Although it may seem that women are less daring than men, this is not a natural gender characteristic. Most of the time, daring women are called "reckless" for not controlling their sexual inclinations. As a result, women tend to be more subtly vague when discussing or expressing their thoughts on their goals, fantasies, and desires. They merely require a companion who will listen to them!

Orgasms are not important to women

This is a reasonably egotistical myth that should be dispelled. Women still engage in sexual activity without orgasm, but that does not diminish its significance. Although most women find it challenging to orgasm just through penetration, many other ways exist. It will help spice things up with foreplay! Women would appreciate it if their spouses put forth a bit more effort to assist them in obtaining one.

Taboos and fears among larger communities, friends and family, and even women themselves pose obstacles to women's welfare. All people need to have good sexual and reproductive health, yet cisgender and transgender women and girls around the world face numerous challenges to achieving this. Women can have an active and positive sexual life without experiencing physical or mental suffering when they can access open-ended conversations.

The above-discussed points clearly show how biased the assumptions and perspectives are. The motive was not to highlight the ongoing issues but to put a spotlight on why so many people have unsatisfied sexual life, why men are inferior, why men fail to understand what their women want and how men & women are being brainwashed which is ruining the main essence of their life. Sexual activity is an intense, emotional and intimate act wherein it requires two individuals to be involved on the same level. Still, a concept of taboo makes one of the partners less active or participate in the act with a mindset to serve. When so-called taboos are eliminated, healthy sex lives exist. When women understand them better, they will be a better sexual partner, not an object of sex. When men know a women's desires, they would be men in the actual sense. The concept of sex is such a broad term which allows individuals to explore, understand each other and keep the spark and love alive and there is no shame in accepting it with an open mind.

Chapter 8
Good Sex Vs Bad Sex

Sexual activity is timeless, hot, and lovely. The thrilling moment of having an intimate relationship with your spouse can't truly be put into words. Although physical intimacy and sex can play a significant role in partnerships When it comes to sex in a relationship, don't try to find a one-size-fits-all solution; you can still have a solid, healthy relationship, regardless of how much sex you share. Many people—including asexuals and those with low libidos—enjoy deep and lasting partnerships without utilizing sex as a fundamental component. Many others—including those who require frequent sexual engagement for a good love relationship—cannot. Whether it's physical intimacy or not, it's essential to understand the concept of good sex and bad sex.

What is Good Sex

When you let sex happen organically, it's good sex. When you pay attention to your body rather than scheduling romance on a calendar. Living in the present is the key to having good sex. When you're not looking at the time every five seconds, hoping it will soon be over so you won't miss the show's start or be late for work. When you let things happen naturally rather than becoming sidetracked by all the other things you could be doing, open communication is the key to having good sex. When you're both at ease with each other, good sex happens. When you're confident, you have good sex because your spouse keeps staring at you like you're the hottest thing in the universe.

Characteristics of Good Sex

- Sex should not be hurting

A "typical" level of discomfort would be a slight pang or a brief moment of friction that disappears soon with position modifications or the continuation of sex. Penetrative sex is not always pain-free, and persistent or recurring pain is unnatural. Do not disregard pain experienced during intercourse. Pain from sex reduces your capacity to enjoy sex and might impact your libido or desire to have sex again. It is abuse if you complain about discomfort while having sex and your partner doesn't stop. Don't hesitate to ask for help.

- **Both partners have an orgasm**

Absolutely, not everyone is going to have an orgasmic experience every time they have sex. In general, women require more foreplay to experience orgasms. Some women may be reluctant to request more foreplay to enjoy sex, especially in new relationships, and some partners may not be aware of how much foreplay their partner may require to climax. If you pretend to be having fun, your partner might never figure out what makes you climax. You should be able to discuss our sexual happiness, orgasms, and expectations in a healthy partnership.

- **Open communication and setting the boundaries**

You should be aware of your partner's sexual inclinations, and they should be mindful of yours. Every one of us has the right to set and acknowledge appropriate boundaries. When someone crosses limits that have been explicitly stated, it indicates that both your relationship and your sex life are toxic.

- **The frequency is satisfactory to both couples**

Most partnerships begin with more frequent sex. This alters as we have kids, go through stressful times, or our partners experience health issues. That frequency resumes when we feel connected to our relationships, are in good physical and mental health, and are content with our lives. What matters most is that both spouses feel comfortable discussing their expectations and can reach an amicable solution.

- **There is a connection outside the bedroom**

We frequently become comfortable in our relationships. We adore our relationships but switch to autopilot mode and become roommates. To strengthen the bond, we must take the relationship off "autopilot". Spend the night away from home together. Once in a time, initiate closeness. Your spouse may start to feel the effects if they are the only ones making the first move and are consistently rejected. Make a concerted effort to initiate regularly, hold yourself accountable, and build a connection outside the bedroom.

What is bad sex

In recent years, "bad sex" has become a catchphrase to

describe how sex can still be about bad touch and is often non-consensual. Nonetheless, there are other ways to define terrible sex, including lack of orgasm, pain, discomfort, or boredom from staring at the ceiling. The intensity of on-screen sex is rarely matched in real-life sexual encounters, and Real-world sex isn't flawless and doesn't always have a dramatic conclusion. We receive little, if any, education regarding what constitutes a good and healthy sex life, and our sex education focuses more on teaching us what to avoid than what to do. How can you tell when your sex life needs extra care?

Characteristics of bad sex

- **Sex seems like another chore**

When something starts to feel like a chore, it's most likely because we've mentally transformed it into one. Sex is supposed to appear like an immensely sexy affair that occurs naturally every single time due to how our media portrays it, which it most certainly can be. Each person is satisfied with their desired requirement. But here's what society and the media don't tell us: Sex involves a ton of communication, intentionality, planning, and messiness. When you start feeling like this, it's a red flag, and you should communicate with your partner to maintain a healthy sex life.

- **You're not a huge fan of sex**

You've read about it in novels and movies, and your pals can't seem to stop talking about it, but you have no sexual desire at all. If you're not experiencing any pleasure, you or your spouse may not be doing well in bed. Don't hesitate to ask for help and identify the problem.

- **You immediately envision penetration when you hear the word "sex"**

Sex is not just about penetration; many think it is like this because of social conditioning. If you believe sex means reaching only the orgasm, it's not true; a lot comes under the umbrella of sex. For some people who have experienced sexual trauma, sex can include personal touch and snuggling. Others consider masturbation as just as much sex as penetrative intercourse with a partner because they are both forms of sexual expression.

- **You experience embarrassment over your sexuality**

You feel uneasy around sex for some reason. When your lover complements you sexually, you feel embarrassed. If you're too preoccupied with what makes a man and woman terrible in bed. In any case, sex causes you much too much stress, and you believe it isn't worth it.

- **You must usually plot out the entire act before performing it**

You prefer to know what's going to happen next. When you know you're going to have sex, you try to organize everything and make sure your partner follows through. At first, this might have seemed hot, but repeating the same two actions makes the process monotonous in bed, and your partner might rapidly grow bored.

- **There is no pillow chat between you and your partner**

The intense sexual encounter ends, and you're done. When your spouse tries to start a conversation after, you show no interest at all. Relationships depend on talking after sex; not talking after sex is a sign that you do not have a good and healthy sex life.

- **You never have foreplay**

You always jump straight in because you believe that foreplay is for losers, and that's a sign you're inexperienced and possibly awful at sex. An excellent method to get things rolling, warm up your partner, and get them interested is through foreplay. A lack of concern for your spouse's feelings can be a tremendous turn-off.

- **You don't have an emotional connection**

Your connection outside the bedroom directly affects how you feel about each other in bed. Your sexual relationship suffers if you don't emotionally connect with your spouse. According to research, if you and your partner don't have an emotional connection, your partner may not feel secure or at ease having sex, which makes it more stressful for both of you.

- **You're being overly assertive**

It might be flattering to express an interest in having sex with your partner but being overly forceful about it can be insulting and may even turn your partner against it.

Tips to improve your sex life

If you have the same feelings for sex, it's evident that we are conditioned to associate sex with guilt, confusion, and insecurity. When discussing sex, people are frequently susceptible. They don't express their likes or dislikes to their partner since they are worried about upsetting them. Yet, you won't get it unless you ask for it. Communicate with your partner, but before you start talking, you should figure out precisely what it is about your sexual life that disturbs you. Is it a matter of technique? Timing? "If you know what isn't working for you, try to rectify the problems. Here are a few tips to transform your bad sex to good and healthy sex life.

1. Develop your sense of confidence

It's time to work on your confidence now that you know how much extremely low or very high confidence can affect how well you perform in bed. If you lack confidence, gradually increase it by employing affirmation strategies, such as thinking well of yourself or participating in activities that will boost your self-assurance.

2. Practice communication skills in bed

Many believe sex is merely a physical act, which is entirely false. Communicating during sex is essential. Scientists also claim that you can communicate with your spouse during sex by using nonverbal signs. You can also try probing your partner about their comfortable and uncomfortable posture preferences. Talking it out will help you improve in bed and convince your lover that you are not a lousy bed partner.

3. Experiment with new stuff

Your lover becomes bored if you only have one bedtime routine. Also, a partner who seems bored with you is a clue that he believes you are not into the act. Change things up. Experiment with foreplays and roleplaying. Take it a step further by asking your partner about their wildest desire. To put it another way, try something new.

4. Make an emotional connection

It is critical to repair your connection outside of the bedroom. A strong emotional connection will help you surpass pointless sex and make your partner's sex more enjoyable. Go on dates and discover a shared interest; perhaps you both enjoy theme parks or binge-watching shows. Other than sex, doing things with your partner can actually help things in the bedroom.

5. Try Foreplay

Foreplay is a sometimes-forgotten aspect of sex. You shouldn't assume your partner is awake and ready to go even when feeling sassy. It's critical to judge your partner's sexual interest, and a little foreplay can help you improve in bed. It can also help you and your spouse relax if you are uncomfortable and assist both of you in developing chemistry.

6. You can try therapy

It may sound over the top, but attending sex therapy can improve your effectiveness in bed. Sex therapists can assist you in identifying any issues you may be having and their possible causes. If your partner is the one who has a problem with sex, going to therapy sessions together can help you develop a stronger bond, solve issues in your relationships, both inside and outside the bedroom, and make sex more enjoyable for you as you date.

7. Have an open communication

Take the initiative and ask: What do you prefer in the bedroom? What about my body do you like? How do you feel in a particular position? These are some conversation starters you can ask your partner. Consider turning it into a game if talking about it makes you feel awkward or uncomfortable. There are also many couples dating questions available online. It doesn't have to be a serious discussion; focus on being more comfortable chatting openly about sex. It's nothing to be embarrassed about!

8. Start slow

Many believe that taking things slowly indicates that you're lousy at sex, a widespread misunderstanding. Slowing down might make sex more enjoyable for you and your partner by making it more exciting. It also allows you and your companion to become acquainted with one another.

9. Be spontaneous

A normal relationship can rapidly become monotonous, affecting your effectiveness in bed. Be adventurous and impulsive. Take your partner on a surprise date or overnight getaway. Being impulsive can excite your relationship and give you more energy and vigor in bed.

Being unsatisfactory in bed is not an irrevocable verdict; it is a skill that must be developed, just like any other. You can improve your sex life by communicating openly with your partner, attempting new things in the bedroom, and focusing on your own self-confidence. Attending sex therapy or counseling is another excellent technique to improve your sexual life. Don't stress out and enjoy every second of the experience, don't focus on the mind-blowing orgasm. Good sex is about not regretting a minute of your time spent with your partner and looking forward to enjoying it all over again.

Good Sex Tips for Senior Sex

Sex can be an intense emotional experience and a valuable tool for protecting or improving health, and it's not only for teenagers. There will always be a craving for intimacy. And current research supports the idea that you can indulge in sex for as long as you choose, regardless of gender. Sex at 70 or 80 is undoubtedly different from that at 20 or 30, but it can also be better in some respects. Emotional difficulties can alter sexual feelings at any age. This isn't always bad news. Many older couples report having better sex lives because they have fewer distractions, more time and solitude, and no pregnancy anxieties. On the other hand, some adults may be stressed out due to health issues, financial difficulties, or other lifestyle changes. Your desire for sex may decrease due to depression.

What changes can be anticipated?

One's mental and physical well-being frequently influences sexuality. What you can accomplish depends on how you feel physically, and what you want to do depends on how you feel emotionally. Many elderly couples are more satisfied with their sex life than when they were younger. They may have fewer distractions, more leisure and privacy, and no concerns about pregnancy. They could also communicate their needs and wants more effectively, leading to closer closeness and connection opportunities.

Physical changes that come with aging are also common, and they can occasionally make it difficult to engage in and enjoy sex. Our bodies, including our weight, skin, and muscular tone, change as we age. Some older adults are dissatisfied with their aging bodies and might be concerned that they won't be as desirable to their lovers anymore. Physical problems caused by health ailments, stress, and concern can obstruct intimacy and a fulfilling sex life.

There are many changes, but it doesn't mean that you seniors can't enjoy sex; here are a few tips that will help to enjoy sex as it's a part of human life.

- **Communication**

A lot more factors contribute to intimacy than just the act of having sex. It all begins with communication and a willingness to discuss significant concerns between partners. It is also critical in addressing trust issues, unresolved disputes, and a lack of connection with one another. Our attitudes toward sex may also alter as we age due to internal conflicts, such as low self-esteem or a persistent health problem. Communicate with each other and discuss all your insecurities and wants.

- **Give time to yourself**

Your sexual arousal decreases with age. To increase your chances of success, you and your partner should look for a place for sex that is peaceful, relaxing, and free from distractions. Moreover, be aware that it will take you longer to become aroused and have an orgasm due to the physical changes to your body. Spending more time having sex isn't necessarily bad; including these physical demands in your lovemaking routine can open the door to a new sexual encounter.

- **Exercise regularly**

Exercise is a great mood booster and keeps your body in shape. Physical activity increases the release of serotonin, resulting in good sentiments that are beneficial to sexual desire. When they're down and out, few people feel aroused. As you might expect, having sex can be exercise, which benefits the heart and brain. A healthy sexual life is associated with a lower incidence of heart disease and prostate cancer in males. Sex can lessen incontinence in older women and strengthen the pelvic muscles.

- **Don't hesitate to use lubrication.**

Females often need a little help from water-based lubricants as they age because their natural lubrication for sexual activity tends to decline. Sex without adequate lubrication can cause significant discomfort and vaginal injury. Although they are usually utilized during sexual activity, lubricants can also be used topically to moisten the vagina.

- **Think beyond intercourse**

There are alternative ways to experience intimacy and pleasure if you or your spouse can no longer do this. Kissing and touching are basic but intimate activities that should not be disregarded. You and your companion should also consider offering sensual massages to one another, oral sex, and experimenting with sex items such as vibrators.

We are so secretive about sex after the age of 50. One primary reason is that sexual health is taboo; as we avoid discussing a topic, it can become riddled with myths and preconceptions. Physical changes frequently result in less intense responses during middle and older age than young sex. But, the emotional byproducts of maturity — greater self-assurance, improved communication abilities, and lower levels of inhibition — can contribute to developing a deeper, more complex, and ultimately rewarding sexual encounter. A crucial aspect of getting older is maintaining your sexual health. You may increase your chances of having a long and good sex life by staying healthy, tackling challenges gently, and communicating openly with your spouse.

Chapter 9
A Healthy Sex Life

These days, we are overloaded with information regarding our romantic lives. It's everywhere; if you pick a newspaper, magazine, or social media, there is plenty of information from the newest techniques to satisfy your lover, satisfy yourself, be more adventurous in bed, reap more health advantages from sex, and be more connected and in love with your relationship. The sexual revolution seems to have created a culture where everyone privately worries about how they are doing or if their sex life is healthy or not.

What is Healthy Sex Life?

How frequently you engage in sex or even experience, orgasms are not the main focus of a healthy sexual life. Intimacy is key to excellent sex; occasionally, a decent massage or holding each other can suffice. Instead, this kind of contact can enhance sexual chemistry, a crucial aspect of intimacy. Being indulging in healthy sex means being able to:

- Talk openly about your emotions and principles.
- Decide whether to initiate or refuse sex.

- Experience climax, excitement, and sexual expression without embarrassment, shame, or guilt.
- Use your sexual freedom.

Healthy sexuality includes not only your gender but also your:

- Emotions, physical needs, and attitudes.
- Bodily and emotional needs.
- Throughout your life, you will have sexual demands and desires.
- Enjoyment and satisfaction.
- Respect for oneself.

Characteristics of Healthy Sexual Relationships

- **One feels better after having sex**

In a good sexual relationship, one feels security, connection, and affirmation. The patience and determination required to overcome feelings of threat, alienation, and shame will be rewarded.

- **Feelings, Both Emotional and Physical**

Both parties in a happy intimate relationship are conscious of their physical and emotional sensations. There is no need for numbing agents or "chasing the orgasm" while experiencing them favorably.

- **The Rediscovery of Passion and Creativity**

This isn't only restricted to sexual activity; it could also involve rediscovering genuine creative pursuits like music, painting, or writing. Sex is no longer the main channel for emotional expression.

- **You care for yourself in ways other than sexual**

If you consistently and purposefully engage in other forms of pleasure, your experience of healthy sexuality will be more authentic. Healthy sexuality is not the only avenue for self-nurturance. Enjoy sensuous physical pursuits like dancing in the rain, taking a hot bubble bath, or sipping a warm cup of tea.

- **You Have the Potential to Be Emotionally Vulnerable**

A healthy personal relationship makes you recognize that vulnerability is essential to relate honestly with people, unlike sex addicts who sexualize their sentiments to insulate themselves from vulnerability out of fear of betrayal.

- **Balanced and moderate sexuality exists**

As you reach sexual maturity, you can control an appropriate flow of sexual energy, unlike others who live in the extremes of sexual energy, experiencing either full-on overwhelming sexual tension or repressed, walled-off sexual impulses.

Benefits of Healthy Sex Life

Healthy sex life can provide several emotional and physical benefits given below

Emotional Benefits

Stress reliever: You feel joyful when you have consenting sex with a caring partner. You can vacation from your daily concerns by engaging in sexual activity. It is a comfort to get a break, even if it is only for an hour.

Understanding each other feelings: A fulfilling, healthy sexual relationship strengthens intimacy between partners. Your everyday partnership with your partner encourages both trust and compassion.

Healthy Libido: You've probably heard the saying, "Use it or lose it". Regular sexual engagement is consistent with this. Moreover, women are physiologically more able to engage in sexual activity and orgasm regularly.

Physical Benefits

There are many motives to engage in sexual activity. Some of the most frequent explanations for having sex include recreation, emotional well-being, companionship, and conception. It's time to include "for health reasons" to the list. Several health advantages will come to you as a result of having a healthy sexual life:

An immunity booster: Sexual activity increases the production of immune-fighting antibodies when it occurs regularly, once or twice weekly. This aids your body's ability to fight off sickness.

A happy heart: Making love not only makes you joyful, but it may also prevent men and women from heart disease. It causes an increase in heart rate. Sex is comparable to exercise. Yet, it also balances testosterone and estrogen hormones in men and women, which are essential for heart health.

Blood pressure reduction: Exercise and happiness together can reduce blood pressure. Sexual intercourse accomplishes this.

Gender-specific benefits: Ejaculation has been found to reduce men's risk of developing prostate cancer. Sexual activity helps women's bladders strengthen, enhancing bladder performance. Moreover, regular sex helps lubricate a woman's vagina. In particular, as people get older, it is more pleasant for women to have sex.

Sound Sleep: Prolactin is a hormone that your body immediately starts to generate following an orgasm. In addition, oxytocin is a hormone released during orgasm by both men and women that encourages sound sleep.

Harmful Effects of Sexual Scoring

In layman's language, sexual scoring focuses on the number of sexual partners a person has, especially a man. Regarding sexuality and sex, there are different rules for men and women. We see women as timid, and when a woman makes a sexual relationship with more than one partner, she is labeled as characterless. However, for men, one key component of "being a man" in society is having sex with different partners.

Let's be clear—having much sex or being straight are both perfectly acceptable. Yet, if men base their self-worth and value on how much sex they engage in to ensure they are engaging in enough sex to maintain their "manhood," we have a problem.

It creates circumstances in which males feel pushed to have sex, even when they don't want to, and it plays a significant role in why men resort to the coercion of both verbal and physical kinds to acquire sex from women. That is why this convention is so ubiquitous and harmful: it normalizes a culture in which males are expected to do anything to have sex. It turns sex into a game where the object is to score more points at the expense of the women, who are made into targets or challenges to be overcome.

"Boys will be boys", These kinds of comments promote and justify this standard, which causes many men to always feel under pressure to outdo one another. It encourages men to prove their masculinity with heterosexual sex. Since men always have to want and enjoy sex, it's assumed they can't be the victim. Men are victims of maintaining false manhood norms, and gender-based violence is normalized.

Keeping scores in sexual life is not a healthy relationship with yourself. There is much more to having good sexual health than just engaging in safe sex or being able to get intimate. Sexual health refers to your perception of yourself as a sexual being, your capacity to embrace and enjoy your sexuality, and your feeling that you own your sexual behavior and preferences. Big-time pleasure comes from having a healthy sexual life. Furthermore, satisfying, healthy sex is essential to your health and well-being. Sex, especially an orgasm, can improve mood, promote sleep, relax you, and even lower pain by releasing oxytocin, endorphins, and other feel-good chemicals in the brain.

Chapter 10

Sex Life During & After Pregnancy

When a baby enters your life, your thoughts in bed are most likely very different from before. The bedroom was most likely your calm, relaxed, serene area and where you might have displayed your sexuality. Many of these things, however, may feel far away with a newborn. This will alter over time. Your body will recover, and you'll grow more at ease in your new job as a parent. Your ideas will eventually shift from "Let's get some sleep" to "Let's get physical".

There are many do's and don't's when it comes to sex during and after pregnancy. Let's find out if it is safe to have sex during and after pregnancy.

Sex during pregnancy

A positive pregnancy test can portend significant changes in your sexual life over the ensuing nine months. Sex can indeed feel different during pregnancy than before, from figuring out which sex positions feel comfortable with an expanding belly to navigating sensations like nausea and breast pain. But it doesn't mean you must put your love-making sessions on hold!

It's possible that having sex while pregnant will feel different from having it previously. Hormones and increased blood flow to your genitals during pregnancy might make sex pleasurable. However, symptoms such as aching breasts, nausea, and an increasing belly can make sex unpleasant. Additionally, it's common to experience brief stomach contractions or cramps during or after intercourse. These cramps could be caused by the contraction of the muscles in your uterus during orgasm. Biological factors in a male partner's semen can also cause cramps. Having sex during pregnancy offers several advantages for both physical and mental health, from reducing stress to fostering close relationships. Furthermore, as long as you don't have any pregnancy issues, it's normally safe to use during all three trimesters. We'll go over why you should continue having sex while pregnant.

Benefits of sex during pregnancy

Sex is a healthful activity that most pregnant women can engage in safely. For many couples, pregnancy sex is crucial and provides both physical and emotional advantages. Here are seven reasons to consider being intimate with your partner for nine months.

Sex during pregnancy fosters connection

Pregnant women frequently become preoccupied with their growing fetuses, excluding their partners. Physical affection can help your relationship grow and make your partner feel important. Later in the pregnancy, post-intercourse cuddling sessions are ideal for your partner to feel the baby kick.

Pregnant sex can be much more pleasurable

Some people experience heightened orgasms because pregnancy increases blood flow to the pubic area, boosting sensitivity. More estrogen makes your vagina moist and may cause your breasts to be more sensitive. These physical alterations frequently combine to produce fantastic sex for many people, which is not the case for everyone. To have successful and satisfying prenatal sex, you and your partner must determine what works and feels appropriate.

Stress reliever

The hormone oxytocin, released during an orgasm and causes endorphin production, floods your body, making you feel relaxed and content. When stressed out, remember that having sex releases endorphins, which can help you feel more comfortable and even lessen discomfort. Furthermore, the distraction of sex can help you forget about your pregnancy worries!

Sexual activity sharpens your sense of body

Allowing yourself time for sexual pleasure and connection, whether with a partner or alone, will enable you to calm down and tune into your body. Pay attention to and enjoy all the extraordinary bodily changes as your pregnancy advances. What more enjoyable method to take in this period than with sensual touch? Love your body and be amazed by the strength and beauty of childbirth.

Sex is good for your mental health

A fulfilling sex life delivers a long-term benefit to your mental health and the immediate high that comes from having sex. Regular sex has been shown to boost your mood and quality of life.

Sex can ease labor and recovery

Your pelvic muscles tighten when you have an orgasm, making them stronger. This facilitates bladder control throughout pregnancy, lessens the intensity of labor contractions, and might hasten postpartum recovery. Of course, you can do Kegels in between sex sessions as well!

If your doctor hasn't advised you otherwise, having sex while pregnant is completely safe. It is typical for your sexual desire to shift during pregnancy. This isn't cause for concern, but discussing it with your sexual partner can assist. You may enjoy having sex when pregnant, or you may not want to. You can find alternative ways to love or make love. The most important thing is to express your emotions to your mate. There are many myths related to sex during pregnancy; let's debunk them.

Myths regarding sex during pregnancy

Myth 1: Deep Penetration Can Be Harmful to the Baby

Fact: This is a massive myth. You probably aren't aware that during sex, your vagina stretches. The penis and cervix naturally separate by a few centimeters, and the cervix is closed and sealed with a thick mucus plug to safeguard the infant. Additionally, the baby is lying in the amniotic sac, which was created to keep them snug and safe inside your uterus.

Myth 2: Contractions caused by orgasm can result in a miscarriage

Fact: Those minor cramps you may experience following sex are entirely normal; they result from the uterus' muscles contracting slightly. As long as you are not carrying a high-risk pregnancy, they won't harm you. The contractions you experience during and after orgasm are not the type that would result in a miscarriage. There are two different types of contractions. Don't confuse these moderate contractions with labor contractions, which will be unpleasant and occur at regular intervals every three to five minutes.

Myth 3: Pregnant sex hurts

Fact: Certain positions will be off-limits since they may cause you discomfort, but many individuals find pregnant sex to be more delightful than ordinary sex. This is due to engorged genitals and more sensitive nerve endings. Furthermore, oxytocin, a hormone that increases during pregnancy, fuels feelings of lust. Some even have their first orgasms while pregnant.

Myth 4: Different postures can affect the sex of the baby

Fact: The baby's sex is determined once the sperm and egg have mated. The baby will be a girl if the sperm fertilizes; the egg has an X chromosome. The baby will be a male if the sperm contains a Y chromosome. There has been no established effect of sex influence on sexual posture before or after pregnancy.

When sex during pregnancy is not good?

Sometimes, you may have to forego specific activities

or positions or stop having sex for a portion of your pregnancy. Your ob-gyn will inform you if you have - or develop - any issues that make sex impossible. Your doctor may advise you not to have sex if you have the following:

- Early birth (or a history of premature labor)
- Vaginal bleeding or discharge that is not explained
- Inadequate cervical function
- Before the third trimester, a dilated cervix
- Membranes that have ruptured (your water has broken)
- A genital herpes outbreak (or oral herpes if you're having oral sex) or Other sexually transmitted infections (STIs)

Most women report that sex feels different throughout their pregnancy. It may be more pleasurable sometimes, but you may not enjoy it or feel up to it at others. Sex during pregnancy may also feel different due to specific anatomical changes. The sensation that may heighten your sex-related enjoyment might be brought on by increased blood flow to the pelvic area. You may experience more natural vaginal lubrication, which could be beneficial. On the other hand, more sensitivity in specific locations may feel uncomfortable or unpleasant during pregnant sex. In addition, although they are not unusual, you can have a few tiny stomach cramps or contractions during or right after an orgasm.

Hence, sex during pregnancy can be a different experience, but always tell your partner if anything about sex makes you uncomfortable.

Sex after Pregnancy

Pregnancy and childbirth alter your body as well as

your sexual life significantly. Hormonal changes after birth may cause vaginal tissue to shrink and become more sensitive. Your vaginal, uterine, and cervix must also "return" to standard size. Furthermore, Breastfeeding can reduce libido. In short, your body requires some rest following delivery. There is no set period after childbirth during which you must refrain from having sex. However, most doctors advise women to wait four to six weeks after a vaginal delivery.

How does giving birth affect sex?

Sex after giving birth will feel different. According to research, 83 percent of females suffered sexual issues in the first three months after their first delivery. However, as the post-pregnancy months pass, that figure continues to fall.

The following are the most typical problems with sex after delivery:

- Perineal tear or episiotomy bleeding pain
- loose muscles
- vaginal dryness
- weak vaginal tissue, lack of flexibility in vaginal tissue

Hormones are important in postpartum healing and the return to regular sexual activity. Estrogen levels return to pre-pregnancy levels in the days following childbirth, and Breastfeeding may cause estrogen levels to fall below pre-pregnancy levels. Low estrogen levels make vaginal dryness more likely since the hormone produces natural vaginal lubrication. During intercourse, dry tissue can cause irritation and even bleeding, increasing your chances of infection.

Tips for enjoying healthy sex life post-pregnancy

You can have a healthy, joyful sex life after giving birth. These suggestions may be helpful:

- **Take your time**: Your body may not be ready to resume pre-pregnancy activities in the first few weeks after you've been cleared for sex. Take each day as it comes. Massage and other intimate activities can help you warm up to sex again.
- **Increase your foreplay:** Allow enough time for your vagina to produce its own natural lubrication. Before having intimate intercourse, that is, deep penetration, extend foreplay, try mutual masturbation, or do anything else.
- **Apply lubrication:** You may require some assistance as your hormones adjust. Look for a water-based product. Condoms can be damaged, and delicate tissue irritated by oil-based lubes.
- **Exercise Kegels:** Kegel exercises to aid in rebuilding pelvic floor muscles. This can help with typical postpartum concerns such as incontinence. Exercising your muscles can also help you regain vaginal strength and feeling. Longer holds will help you gain stamina.
- **Schedule time for sex: You** and your partner may not have much time for spontaneity with a new baby in the house—schedule time to spend together on your calendars. You won't feel rushed or stressed this way.
- **Communicate with your partner:** Sex after delivery is different but not consistently awful. Others might be exciting and entertaining, but you should retain an open line of communication with your partner about what

feels good and what doesn't. This will allow you to enjoy sex again while eliminating any unnecessary pain.

For a short time, your sexual impulses and experiences may differ from what you recall. That is also perfectly normal. "There are going to be things that work and things that may not". The quality of your experience—and likely theirs—depends on how carefully and thoughtfully you interact with your partner and how well you communicate with them about what's working and what isn't, especially the first few times you attempt. It depends on your physical and mental preparedness when you're "ready-ready" to have sex after giving birth. Pay attention to your body and discuss any concerns with your doctor. Initially, sex might not be what you recall, but with persistence and time, you'll establish a new normal.